A book by   **Cara Gray MS, RD, CDN**

PLANT-BASED
LOW-FODMAP

DIET COOKBOOK

D1716326

CONTENT

INTRODUCTION

Combining a plant-based diet with a low FODMAP diet is known as a plant-based low FODMAP diet. A class of carbohydrates known as FODMAPs—fermentable oligosaccharides, disaccharides, monosaccharides, and polyols—can have a negative impact on how well food is absorbed in the small intestine. Particularly in those with illnesses like irritable bowel syndrome (IBS) or other digestive disorders, they can produce digestive symptoms like bloating, gas, stomach discomfort, and diarrhea.

On the other side, a plant-based diet emphasizes the consumption of complete, unprocessed plant foods while limiting or omitting animal products. It places a focus on foods like fruits, vegetables, grains, legumes, nuts, and seeds since they are full of fiber, healthy plant chemicals, and important nutrients. Numerous health advantages, such as better digestion, a lower risk of chronic diseases, and greater general wellbeing, have been linked to plant-based diets.

Researchers at Monash University came up with the low FODMAP diet, which entails temporarily cutting out or reducing high FODMAP foods from the diet and then gradually returning them to find personal triggers. With the aid of this method, people can pinpoint which specific FODMAPs may be to blame for their digestive issues, tailor their diet accordingly, and successfully control their symptoms.

Given that numerous high FODMAP items, including various fruits, vegetables, legumes, and grains, are frequently available in plant-based sources, combining a plant-based diet with the low FODMAP strategy can be difficult. However, a well-balanced and nutrient-dense plant-based low FODMAP diet is doable with careful planning and item selection.

People can eat a variety of plant-based meals while successfully managing their digestive problems by adhering to a plant-based low FODMAP diet. They are able to benefit from both strategies, which include better digestion, more nutrient absorption, and greater general health and wellbeing.

This cookbook combines these two dietary approaches, providing a wide range of flavorful recipes that are rich in plant-based ingredients while also being low in FODMAPs. It offers guidance on identifying high and low FODMAP foods, pantry essentials, and cooking techniques specific to this style of cooking.

The recipes provided include diverse and creative options for breakfast, brunch, appetizers, snacks, soups, salads, main courses, side dishes, desserts, and beverages. These recipes incorporate low FODMAP fruits, vegetables, grains, legumes, and plant-based protein sources, ensuring a balanced and satisfying plant-based eating experience while supporting digestive health.

WHAT ARE FODMAPS

FODMAP stands for fermentable oligo-, di-, monosaccharides and polyols. These short-chain carbs are resistant to digestion. Instead of being absorbed into your bloodstream, they reach the far end of your intestine, where most of your gut bacteria reside. Your gut bacteria then use these carbs for fuel, producing hydrogen gas and causing digestive symptoms in sensitive individuals. FODMAPs also draw liquid into your intestine, which may cause diarrhea.

Although not everyone has a sensitivity to FODMAPs, it is very common among people with irritable bowel syndrome (IBS).

Common FODMAPs include:

• Fructose: a simple sugar found in many fruits and vegetables that also makes up the structure of table sugar and most added sugars

• Lactose: a carbohydrate found in dairy products like milk

• Fructans: found in many foods, including grains like wheat, spelt, rye and barley

• Galactans: found in large amounts in legumes

• Polyols: sugar alcohols like xylitol, sorbitol, maltitol, and mannitol. They are found in some fruits and vegetables and often used as sweeteners

It Effects on Digestion

The majority of FODMAPs pass through most of your intestine unchanged. They're completely resistant to digestion and are categorized as a dietary fiber.

But some carbs function like FODMAPs only in some individuals. These include lactose and fructose. General sensitivity to these carbs also differs between people. In fact, scientists believe that they contribute to digestive conditions like IBS. When FODMAPs reach your colon, they get fermented and used as fuel by gut bacteria. The same happens when dietary fibers feed your friendly gut bacteria, which leads to various health benefits. However, the friendly bacteria tend to produce methane, whereas the bacteria that feed on FODMAPs produce hydrogen, another type of gas. This may lead to gas, bloating, stomach cramps, pain, and constipation..

Many of these symptoms are caused by distention of the gut, which can also make your stomach look bigger. FODMAPs are also osmotically active, which means that they can draw water into your intestine and contribute to diarrhea.

In some individuals, FODMAPs are poorly digested, so they end up reaching the colon. They draw water into the intestine and get fermented by hydrogen-producing gut bacteria.

Benefits of a plant-based diet for managing digestive issues

The relationship between a plant-based diet and the low FODMAP diet involves adapting plant-based principles while managing FODMAP intake to suit individual needs. It requires careful ingredient selection, recipe modification, and attention to nutritional balance to ensure both dietary approaches are effectively integrated.

A plant-based diet can offer several benefits for managing digestive issues, including the following:

1. High Fiber Content: Plant-based diets are typically rich in dietary fiber, which plays a crucial role in maintaining a healthy digestive system. Fiber adds bulk to the stool, promotes regular bowel movements, and helps prevent or alleviate constipation. It also acts as a prebiotic, providing nourishment for beneficial gut bacteria, which supports a healthy gut microbiome.

2. Anti-inflammatory Properties: Many plant-based foods, such as fruits, vegetables, whole grains, and legumes, are naturally rich in antioxidants and phytonutrients. These compounds have anti-inflammatory properties that can help reduce inflammation in the gastrointestinal tract, providing relief from conditions like inflammatory bowel disease (IBD) or gastritis.

3. Lower Fat Content: Plant-based diets are generally lower in saturated fats and cholesterol compared to diets that include animal products. High-fat foods, especially those high in saturated fats, can be harder to digest and may exacerbate

digestive symptoms. Choosing plant-based fats, such as avocados, nuts, and seeds, can provide healthier fats that are easier on the digestive system.

4. Reduced Irritants: Animal products, particularly red meat and processed meats, have been associated with increased inflammation and digestive discomfort in some individuals. Plant-based diets, which exclude or minimize animal products, may help reduce the consumption of potential irritants and trigger foods, leading to improved digestive comfort.

5. Improved Gut Microbiome: Plant-based diets have been linked to a more diverse and beneficial gut microbiome. A diverse gut microbiome is associated with better digestion, nutrient absorption, and overall gut health. By consuming a variety of plant foods, individuals can promote the growth of beneficial gut bacteria, which can help regulate digestion and support a healthy gut environment.

6. Weight Management: Digestive issues can sometimes be associated with weight management challenges. Plant-based diets, when focused on whole, unprocessed foods, tend to be lower in calories and can support weight management efforts. Maintaining a healthy weight can positively impact digestive health by reducing the risk of conditions like acid reflux, gallstones, and fatty liver disease.

Basics of the low FODMAP diet + Guidelines

A diet low in FODMAPs is essentially a type of elimination diet. Often, a low FODMAP diet is implemented as a healing protocol for irritable bowel syndrome (IBS) or to treat small intestinal bacterial overgrowth (SIBO).

A low FODMAP diet is a 3-step approach to healing digestive issues that includes elimination and reduction, reintroduction, and personalisation.

Other elimination diets include allergy elimination diet, keto, paleo, and autoimmune paleo (AIP). The goal of all elimination diets is to first reduce or eliminate specific foods or food groups that might be a culprit for certain reactions and symptoms. Later, you might reintroduce these foods or increase their intake to observe which ones impact you poorly or – in the case of many elimination diets – increase autoimmune markers and flare-ups.

As mentioned above, the low FODMAP protocol is easily divided into three distinct steps.

Step 1. Elimination

The initial introduction to the low FODMAP diet should last 2-6 weeks. The approach is simple, but it definitely requires some research. You simply want to begin by swapping high FODMAP foods with low FODMAP foods. It is best to stick to low FODMAP foods and also eliminate foods in the 'moderate' ranking. During this time, the ideal outcome is that IBS symptoms improve or dissipate. If so, you can proceed with the next step which will help you fine-tune your understanding of which foods are problematic. However, there is a chance that FODMAPs are not exacerbating your symptoms. In this instance, you will need to consider alternative treatment methods.

Step 2. Reintroduction

Next up is the reintroduction phase. The goal is to develop an understanding of specific FODMAP triggers. In order to figure this out, you will reintroduce one carbohydrate group at a time. This is where you will want a good guide as you will need to choose foods that contain just one FODMAP and no others. You will use this food to monitor symptoms for up to three days and determine whether or not it causes an IBS flare or worsens symptoms.

Step 3. Personalisation

This is where you implement semi-permanent changes. In any elimination diet, the goal is to continue on eating as many foods as possible that don't cause adverse side effects so as to best to enjoy life, cooking, and eating! You will get to know which foods are good for a treat and which simply aren't worth it at all. Well-tolerated foods should be focused on and poorly tolerated foods should be avoided or used for FODMAP challenges down the road to observe potential changes.

Tips for incorporating plant-based foods into a low FODMAP lifestyle

Incorporating plant-based foods into a low FODMAP lifestyle can be challenging, but with some tips and strategies, it can be made easier and more enjoyable. Here are some suggestions to help you navigate this approach:

1. Learn FODMAP-Friendly Plant-Based Foods: Familiarize yourself with low FODMAP plant-based foods that you can include in your diet. This includes low FODMAP fruits like berries, oranges, and grapes, as well as vegetables like carrots, bell peppers, and spinach. Legumes like canned lentils and firm tofu can be used as plant-based protein sources. Gluten-free grains like quinoa, rice, and oats can be staples in your meals.

2. Modify Recipes: Adapt your favorite plant-based recipes to make them low FODMAP. Replace high FODMAP ingredients with suitable alternatives. For example, use infused oils (such as garlic-infused oil) instead of onions and garlic for flavoring. Explore new spice blends and herbs to enhance the taste of your dishes.

3. Experiment with Low FODMAP Plant-Based Proteins: While many legumes are high in FODMAPs, there are low FODMAP options available. Experiment with canned lentils, firm tofu, tempeh, or small amounts of chickpeas or canned black beans to include plant-based protein in your meals. Proper portion control and individual tolerance should be considered.

4. Focus on Whole Foods: Emphasize whole, unprocessed plant foods in your meals. Incorporate a variety of low FODMAP vegetables, fruits, grains, and nuts

into your dishes to ensure a diverse nutrient intake. This helps promote overall health and well-being.

5. Pay Attention to Portion Sizes: Even low FODMAP plant-based foods can become high FODMAP if consumed in large quantities. Be mindful of portion sizes and individual tolerance. Working with a registered dietitian specializing in low FODMAP diets can help you determine suitable serving sizes for different foods.

6. Plan Balanced Meals: Ensure your plant-based low FODMAP meals are nutritionally balanced. Include a mix of carbohydrates, proteins, and healthy fats to provide essential nutrients. Incorporate a variety of colorful fruits and vegetables to enhance the nutritional value of your meals.

7. Seek Recipe Inspiration: Look for plant-based low FODMAP recipe resources, such as cookbooks, websites, or apps, to discover new and creative dishes. These resources can provide ideas and guidance on incorporating plant-based ingredients while adhering to a low FODMAP diet.

8. Experiment with Alternative Cooking Techniques: Explore different cooking methods, such as roasting, steaming, grilling, or sautéing, to enhance the flavors and textures of your plant-based dishes. These techniques can help bring out the natural sweetness and flavors of vegetables and make your meals more enjoyable.

ESSENTIALS FOR YOUR PLANT BASED LOW FODMAP PANTRY

1. Gluten-Free Bread: While gluten-free bread isn't exclusively low in FODMAPs, there are plenty of options out there.

2. Gluten-Free All-Purpose Flour: Again, not all gluten-free flours are going to be low FODMAP and not all low FODMAP flours are going to be gluten-free. That being said, a good 1:1 all-purpose flour replacement is worth its weight in gold. Whether you're thickening soups and sauces or whipping up a batch of low FODMAP muffins, this is one pantry staple you'll want to buy in bulk.

3. Gluten-Free Pasta: No matter what kind of diet you're following, pasta is a staple. A bowl of pasta cooked to al-dente and tossed in garlic-infused olive oil makes for a quick but satisfying meal. You can find pasta made from a variety of gluten-free grains and cereals that area also low in FODMAPs. Quinoa pasta (up to 1 cup) can be a delicious low FODMAP option, though you can't go wrong with a good rice noodle (up to 1 cup).

4. Dairy-Free Milk: Whether you're baking or pouring a bowl of low FODMAP cereal, you'll need a good alternative to cow's milk. One option is to simply buy lactose-free milk (up to 1 cup). If you're looking for a lower calorie or vegan-friendly option, soy milk (up to 1 cup) and oat milk (up to 1/8 cup) are worthy of consideration.

5. Nuts and Seeds: Perfect for snacking, toasted nuts and seeds are perfect for stocking in the pantry. Stock up on roasted peanuts for a filling, protein-packed

snack. Pecans (up to 20g) and walnuts (up to 30g) are a must-have for baking, and Brazil nuts (up to 10 nuts) and macadamia nuts (up to 20 nuts) are great if you're looking for something with a little more flavor. You can use chia seeds (up to 2 tablespoons) to make pudding while pumpkin seeds (up to 2 tablespoons) and sunflower seeds (up to 3 tablespoons) make for a salty snack.

6. Dried Herbs and Spices: Any diet becomes instantly more bearable when the food you're enjoying is flavorful. Fill your pantry with low FODMAP herbs like basil, coriander, oregano, and rosemary (all up to 1 cup). Better yet, grab a jar of Italian seasoning. Dried spices like cinnamon, ground cumin, ginger, paprika, and turmeric (all up to 1 tablespoon) are flavorful and versatile. And don't forget the salt and pepper!

7. Sauces and Condiments: If you're looking for a quick and healthy meal, a fresh salad drizzled with low FODMAP dressing is perfect. Sprinkle on some low FODMAP nuts for crunch with sliced cucumber for flavor. Other low FODMAP sauces and condiments to keep on hand include gluten-free soy sauce (up to 2 tablespoons) and pasta sauce. Just remember to check the ingredients when you buy to make sure they're low in FODMAPs.

8. Canned Beans and Legumes: As long as you watch your portions, there are plenty of beans and legumes to include in your low FODMAP diet. These foods are not only rich in fiber and protein, but they're inexpensive and incredibly shelf stable. Just be sure to rotate your stock, refilling pantry shelves from the back so you use the foods that expire earlier first.

9. Canned Tomato Products: Whether you're serving up a pasta dinner or whipping up a batch of homemade chili, canned tomato products (up to 1/2 cup) are definitely a pantry staple. Stock up on diced tomatoes, crushed tomatoes, tomato sauce, and prepared pasta sauces. Just be sure to read the label to check for high FODMAP ingredients like onions and garlic.

10. Infused Oils: Cooking oils like olive oil and sesame oil are always a pantry staple, but when you're following the low FODMAP diet infused oils can be a lifesaver. Garlic and onion are high FODMAP foods, but you can still enjoy the flavor by using garlic or onion-infused oils. You can even make your own!

11. Low FODMAP Grains: Though you might need to avoid traditional staples like wheat, barley, and rye, there are still plenty of low FODMAP alternatives. As an added bonus, if you're also following a gluten-free diet, you'll find that the low FODMAP diet overlaps in this area. Try things like rice (up to 1 cup), millet (up to 1 cup), oats (up to ½ cup), and quinoa (up to ½ cup). Don't forget that there are many versions of rice. From brown rice to jasmine rice, you'll never get bored with all the different tastes and textures.

12. Spreads: If you're feeling snackish but want something a little more satisfying than a handful of peanuts, a sandwich is the perfect solution. Grab a slice of your favorite low FODMAP bread and slather one a low FODMAP spread like peanut butter (up to 2 tablespoons) or almond butter (up to 1 tablespoon) – just be sure to buy natural nut butter free from artificial sweeteners. You can even enjoy

certain jams and marmalades in small servings like strawberry, raspberry, and orange.

13. Low FODMAP Sweeteners: A spoonful of sugar gives your morning coffee a hint of sweetness and it's a staple in home baking. While white sugar and brown sugar (up to 1 tablespoon) are low FODMAP-approved, they're not your only options. Maple syrup (up to 2 tablespoons) is a natural sweetener that works well in many recipes, particularly baked goods where a little extra moisture will be appreciated. You can also try rice malt syrup (up to 1 tablespoon) and small amounts of higher FODMAP sweeteners like honey (up to 1 teaspoon) and molasses (up to 1 teaspoon).

14. Potatoes: While potatoes may not have the same shelf-life as canned beans, they're a great option to keep in your pantry. Mashed potatoes are a family favorite and roasted potatoes make a great side dish for pork and beef. They come in all shapes, sizes, and colors, so you're free to get creative. Just be sure to store them in a paper bag or cardboard box in a cool, dark area of the pantry.

15. Snacks and Crackers: No list of pantry staples would be complete without snacks! Tortilla chips are a must-have for low FODMAP snacking and your local grocery store probably offers a selection of popped corn and rice chips as well.

Allowable and prohibited low FODMAP foods

High FODMAP Foods To Avoid

• Garlic & onions

• All beans & lentils

• Wheat and wheat-based products and rye (in large amounts); gluten-based bread or muffins

• Vegetables: artichokes, asparagus, sugar snap peas and green peas

• Fruit: Watermelon, peaches, apples, cherries, nectarines, pears, mango, avocadoes, dried fruit

• Meat/protein: sausage/processed meat, breaded fish or meat

• Pistachios, cashews and almonds

• Plain cow's milk and yoghurt, ice cream, custard

• Honey and high fructose corn syrup

Low FODMAP Foods To Include

• Protein: Meat, fish, seafood, eggs, tofu, tempeh (fermented soy)

• Most oils and fats, peanuts

• Vegetables (with the exception of onions, artichokes, asparagus, cruciferous family and foods otherwise listed as high FODMAP)

• Fruits: Bananas, melons (with the exception of watermelon), kiwi, grapes, citrus (lime, lemon, grapefruit, etc.)

• Grains: Corn, oatmeal, quinoa, rice

• Dairy: hard cheese, brie, camembert, and feta cheeses, lactose-free milk, ice cream, and/or yoghurt.

• Dark chocolate, maple syrup, rice malt syrup, table sugar

• Sourdough bread in moderation

• Coffee and tea

Breakfast and Brunch

Shrimp & Spinach Quiche

Ingredients

- ¾ cup white whole-wheat flour

- ¾ cup all-purpose flour

- ¼ teaspoon salt

- 2 tablespoons cold butter

- 2 tablespoons sour cream

- 2 tablespoons extra-virgin olive oil

- 2-3 tablespoons ice water

- 2 teaspoons extra-virgin olive oil

- 2 cups diced onions

- 1/8 teaspoon salt plus 1/4 teaspoon, divided

- 2 tablespoons water

- 1 cup finely chopped spinach

- ¾ cup chopped cooked shrimp

- 1 tablespoon chopped fresh oregano

- ½ cup crumbled feta cheese

- 4 large eggs

- 2 large egg whites

- ¾ cup low-fat milk

- ¼ cup sour cream

- ¼ teaspoon freshly ground pepper

Directions

1. To prepare crust: Whisk whole-wheat flour and all-purpose flour with salt in a medium bowl. Cut butter into small pieces; using your fingers, quickly rub the butter into the dry ingredients until smaller but still visible.

2. Add sour cream and oil; toss with a fork to combine with the dry ingredients. Sprinkle 2 tablespoons of ice water over the mixture. Toss with a fork until evenly moist; if the mixture seems dry, add up to 1 more tablespoon water. Knead the dough in the bowl a few times--the mixture may still be a little crumbly--then firmly press into a disk. Cover the bowl with plastic wrap and refrigerate for at least 1 hour.

3. To prepare filling & bake quiche: Preheat oven to 375 degrees F. Coat a 9-inch pie pan with cooking spray.

4. Heat oil in a medium skillet over high heat. Add onions and 1/8 teaspoon salt; cook, stirring frequently, until the onions start to brown, 3 to 5 minutes. Add

water, reduce heat to low and cook, stirring frequently, until the onions are golden brown and very soft, about 15 minutes. Remove from heat and let cool while you roll out the crust.

5. Place the dough on a sheet of parchment or wax paper and roll into a 12- to 13-inch circle, dusting the top with a little flour, as needed. (If chilled more than 1 hour, let the dough stand at room temperature for 5 minutes before rolling.) Place the prepared pie pan upside down in the center of the dough. Holding one hand on top of the pan and the other hand underneath the paper, flip pan and dough over so the dough is lining the pan. Remove the paper and patch any tears in the dough. Trim the crust so it evenly overhangs the edge by about 1 inch, then tuck the edges under at the rim and crimp with your fingers or a fork.

6. Spread the caramelized onions in the bottom of the crust. Layer spinach and shrimp on top of the onions and sprinkle with oregano. Top with cheese. Whisk eggs, egg whites, milk, sour cream, pepper and the remaining 1/4 teaspoon salt in a medium bowl. Pour the mixture into the crust.

7. Bake the quiche until puffed and firm when touched in the center, 40 to 50 minutes. Let cool on a wire rack for 15 minutes. To serve, cut into 8 pieces.

Vegan Freezer Breakfast Burritos

Ingredients

• 2 tablespoons avocado oil, divided

• 1 (14 ounce) package extra-firm water-packed tofu, drained and crumbled

• 2 teaspoons chili powder

• 1 teaspoon ground cumin

• ¼ teaspoon salt

• 1 (15 ounce) can reduced-sodium black beans, rinsed

• 1 cup frozen corn, thawed

• 4 scallions, sliced

• ½ cup prepared fresh salsa

• ¼ cup chopped fresh cilantro

• 6 (8 inch) whole-wheat tortillas or wraps

Directions

1. Heat 1 tablespoon oil in a large nonstick skillet over medium heat. Add tofu, chili powder, cumin and salt; cook, stirring, until the tofu is nicely browned, 10 to 12 minutes. Transfer to a bowl.

2. Add the remaining 1 tablespoon oil to the pan. Add beans, corn and scallions and cook, stirring, until the scallions have softened, about 3 minutes. Return the tofu to the pan. Add salsa and cilantro; cook, stirring, until heated through, about 2 minutes more.

3. If serving immediately, warm tortillas (or wraps), but if freezing do not warm them. Divide the bean mixture among the tortillas, spreading evenly over the bottom third of each tortilla. Roll snugly, tucking in the ends as you go. Serve immediately or wrap each burrito in foil and freeze for up to 3 months.

4. To heat in the microwave: Remove foil, cover with a paper towel and microwave on High until hot, 1 1/2 to 2 minutes.

5. To heat over a campfire: Place foil-wrapped burrito on a cooking grate over a medium to medium-hot fire. Cook, turning once or twice, until steaming hot throughout, 5 to 10 minutes if partially thawed, up to 15 minutes if frozen.

Savory Oatmeal with Cheddar, Collards & Eggs

Ingredients

• 2 tablespoons extra-virgin olive oil, divided

• 2 tablespoons diced shallot

• 2 cups rolled oats (see Tip)

• 4 cups water plus 1/2 cup, divided

- ½ teaspoon salt, divided

- ½ teaspoon ground pepper, divided

- 10 cups chopped collard greens (from 1-2 bunches)

- 2 teaspoons red-wine vinegar

- 1 cup shredded Cheddar cheese

- ¼ cup chipotle salsa, plus more for serving

- 4 large eggs, cooked as desired

Directions

1. Heat 1 tablespoon oil in a large saucepan over medium heat. Add shallot and cook, stirring occasionally, until softened, 1 to 2 minutes. Add oats and stir for 1 minute. Add 4 cups water and 1/4 teaspoon each salt and pepper. Bring to a boil, then reduce heat to a simmer. Cook, stirring often, until creamy, 10 to 12 minutes.

2. Meanwhile, heat the remaining 1 tablespoon oil in a large skillet over medium-high heat. Add collards along with the remaining 1/2 cup water and 1/4 teaspoon each salt and pepper. Cook, stirring occasionally, until tender, 5 to 7 minutes. Remove from heat and stir in vinegar.

3. Stir cheese and salsa into the oatmeal. Serve with the collards, eggs and more salsa, if desired.

Egg in a Hole" Peppers with Avocado Salsa

Ingredients

• 2 bell peppers, any color

• 1 avocado, diced

• ½ cup diced red onion

• 1 jalapeño pepper, minced

• ½ cup chopped fresh cilantro, plus more for garnish

• 2 tomatoes, seeded and diced

• Juice of 1 lime

• ¾ teaspoon salt, divided

• 2 teaspoons olive oil, divided

• 8 large eggs

• ¼ teaspoon ground pepper, divided

Directions

1. Slice tops and bottoms off bell peppers and finely dice. Remove and discard seeds and membranes. Slice each pepper into four 1/2-inch-thick rings.

2. Combine the diced pepper with avocado, onion, jalapeño, cilantro, tomatoes, lime juice, and 1/2 teaspoon salt in a medium bowl.

3. Heat 1 teaspoon oil in a large nonstick skillet over medium heat. Add 4 bell pepper rings, then crack 1 egg into the middle of each ring. Season with 1/8 teaspoon each salt and pepper. Cook until the whites are mostly set but the yolks are still runny, 2 to 3 minutes. Gently flip and cook 1 minute more for runny yolks, 1 1/2 to 2 minutes more for firmer yolks. Transfer to serving plates and repeat with the remaining pepper rings and eggs.

4. Serve with the avocado salsa and garnish with additional cilantro, if desired.

Sheet-Pan Eggs with Spinach & Ham

Ingredients

- 18 large eggs

- ¼ cup reduced-fat milk

- 1 ½ teaspoons smoked paprika

- 1 teaspoon salt

- 1 teaspoon ground pepper

- 1 teaspoon onion powder

- 1 (10 ounce) package frozen chopped spinach, thawed and squeezed dry

- 1 cup shredded sharp Cheddar cheese

- ½ cup diced ham

Directions

1. Preheat oven to 300 degrees F. Generously coat a large rimmed baking sheet with cooking spray.

2. Whisk eggs, milk, smoked paprika, salt, pepper and onion powder together in a large bowl. Pour onto the prepared baking sheet and sprinkle with spinach, Cheddar and ham. Bake until just set, 20 to 25 minutes, rotating the pan from back to front halfway through baking to ensure even cooking. Cut into 12 squares and serve.

Baked Eggs in Tomato Sauce with Kale

Ingredients

• 1 tablespoon extra-virgin olive oil

• 3 10-ounce packages frozen chopped kale, thawed, drained and squeezed dry (9 cups)

• ½ teaspoon salt, divided

• ¼ teaspoon ground pepper, divided

• 1 25-ounce jar low-sodium marinara sauce or 3 cups canned low-sodium tomato sauce

• 8 large eggs

Directions

1. Preheat oven to 350 degrees F.

2. Heat oil in a 10-inch cast-iron skillet or nonstick ovenproof skillet over medium heat. Add kale, season with 1/4 teaspoon salt and 1/8 teaspoon pepper, and sauté for 2 minutes. Stir in marinara (or tomato) sauce and bring to a simmer.

3. Make 8 wells in the sauce with the back of a spoon and carefully crack an egg into each well. Season the eggs with the remaining 1/4 teaspoon salt and 1/8 teaspoon pepper.

4. Transfer the pan to the oven and bake until the egg whites are set and the yolks are still soft, about 20 minutes.

Southwest Breakfast Skillet

Ingredients

• 4 strips center-cut low-sodium bacon (4 ounces)

• 12 ounces Yukon Gold or red potatoes, scrubbed and cut into 1/2-inch pieces

• ¼ cup water, plus more if needed

• 8 ounces white button mushrooms, diced

• 1 medium red, orange or yellow bell pepper, diced

• ½ small red onion, diced

- ¼ teaspoon salt, divided

- ¼ teaspoon ground pepper, divided

- 4 cups Swiss chard, stemmed and thinly sliced (from 1 bunch)

- 1 clove garlic, minced

- 4 large eggs

- ½ cup shredded Cheddar cheese

- ¼ cup chopped fresh cilantro

- ¼ cup prepared salsa or pico de gallo

Directions

1. Cook bacon in a large nonstick skillet over medium heat, flipping once, until crispy, 5 to 7 minutes. Transfer the bacon to a paper-towel-lined plate. Pour off all but 2 teaspoons of the bacon fat.

2. Return the pan to medium heat. Add potatoes and cook, stirring often, for 2 minutes. Add water; cover and steam for 5 minutes, stirring once halfway through. Add mushrooms, bell pepper, onion, and 1/8 teaspoon each salt and pepper; cook, stirring occasionally, until the vegetables are tender, about 5 minutes. Stir in chard and garlic; cook until the chard is tender and wilted, about 2 minutes more. Crumble the bacon and stir into the mixture.

3. Spread the mixture evenly in the pan. Using the back of a wooden spoon, make 4 indentations. Crack 1 egg into each indentation (see Tip). Season with the

remaining 1/8 teaspoon each salt and pepper. Cover and cook until the egg whites are set, about 5 minutes.

4. Remove from heat and top with cheese, cilantro and salsa (or pico de gallo).

Vegan Chickpea Frittata

Ingredients

- 1 cup chickpea flour

- 2 tablespoons nutritional yeast

- 1 teaspoon baking powder

- ½ teaspoon kala namak (black salt) or regular salt (see Tip)

- ¼ teaspoon ground turmeric

- ¼ teaspoon ground pepper

- 1 cup water

- 2 tablespoons lemon juice

- 1 teaspoon reduced-sodium tamari or soy sauce (see Tip)

- 3 teaspoons extra-virgin olive oil, divided

- 1 cup thinly sliced red onion

- 1 cup sliced cremini mushrooms

- 2 teaspoons finely chopped garlic

- 1 cup grape tomatoes, halved lengthwise

- 1 cup packed fresh spinach, roughly chopped

Directions

1. Whisk chickpea flour, nutritional yeast, baking powder, kala namak (or salt), turmeric and pepper together in a medium bowl. Add water, lemon juice and tamari (or soy sauce); whisk until smooth.

2. Heat 1 1/2 teaspoons oil in a medium nonstick skillet over medium heat. Add onion, mushrooms and garlic; cook, stirring occasionally, until the vegetables are soft, 5 to 6 minutes. Add to the chickpea mixture, along with tomatoes and spinach; stir until evenly combined. Do not wipe the pan clean.

3. Add remaining 1 1/2 teaspoons of the oil to the pan; heat over medium heat. Add the chickpea mixture; spread in an even layer. Cover and reduce heat to medium-low; cook, undisturbed, until firm and set, 15 to 20 minutes. Remove from heat. Garnish with chives, if desired.

Chickpea & Potato Hash

Ingredients

- 4 cups frozen shredded hash brown potatoes

- 2 cups finely chopped baby spinach

29

- ½ cup finely chopped onion

- 1 tablespoon minced fresh ginger

- 1 tablespoon curry powder

- ½ teaspoon salt

- ¼ cup extra-virgin olive oil

- 1 15-ounce can chickpeas, rinsed

- 1 cup chopped zucchini

- 4 large eggs

Directions

1. Combine potatoes, spinach, onion, ginger, curry powder and salt in a large bowl.

2. Heat oil in a large nonstick skillet over medium-high heat. Add the potato mixture and press into a layer. Cook, without stirring, until crispy and golden brown on the bottom, 3 to 5 minutes.

3. Reduce heat to medium-low. Fold in chickpeas and zucchini, breaking up chunks of potato, until just combined. Press back into an even layer. Carve out 4 "wells" in the mixture. Break eggs, one at a time, into a cup and slip one into each indentation. Cover and continue cooking until the eggs are set, 4 to 5 minutes for soft-set yolks.

Creamy Scrambled Eggs with Chives

Ingredients

• 2 large eggs

• 1 tablespoon plain kefir

• 2 teaspoons minced chives

• Pinch of salt

• 1 teaspoon butter

Directions

1. Whisk eggs, kefir, chives and salt in a bowl. Add butter to a small skillet over low to medium heat. When the butter has melted, add the egg mixture and scramble with a fork until just set.

Appetizers and Snacks

Almond-Crusted Chicken Fingers

Ingredients

• Canola oil cooking spray

• ½ cup sliced almonds

• ¼ cup whole-wheat flour

• 1 ½ teaspoons paprika

• ½ teaspoon garlic powder

• ½ teaspoon dry mustard

• ¼ teaspoon salt

• ⅛ teaspoon freshly ground pepper

• 1 ½ teaspoons extra-virgin olive oil

• 4 large egg whites

• 1 pound chicken tenders, (see Ingredient Note)

Directions

1. Preheat oven to 475 degrees F. Line a baking sheet with foil. Set a wire rack on the baking sheet and coat it with cooking spray.

2. Place almonds, flour, paprika, garlic powder, dry mustard, salt and pepper in a food processor; process until the almonds are finely chopped and the paprika is mixed throughout, about 1 minute. With the motor running, drizzle in oil; process until combined. Transfer the mixture to a shallow dish.

3. Whisk egg whites in a second shallow dish. Add chicken tenders and turn to coat. Transfer each tender to the almond mixture; turn to coat evenly. (Discard any remaining egg white and almond mixture.) Place the tenders on the prepared rack and coat with cooking spray; turn and spray the other side.

4. Bake the chicken fingers until golden brown, crispy and no longer pink in the center, 20 to 25 minutes.

Italian Turkey Meatballs

Ingredients

• 8 ounces mushrooms, chopped

• 1 small onion, chopped

• 1 stalk celery, sliced

• 4 cloves garlic

• 1 tablespoon extra-virgin olive oil

• ½ cup fine dry breadcrumbs

- ½ cup finely chopped Italian parsley

- ¼ cup grated Parmesan cheese

- 2 teaspoons Italian seasoning

- ½ teaspoon salt

- ½ teaspoon ground pepper

- 1 pound lean ground turkey

Directions

1. Finely chop mushrooms, onion, celery and garlic in a food processor. Heat oil in a large skillet over medium-high heat. Add the vegetable mixture and cook, stirring occasionally, until the liquid has evaporated, 6 to 8 minutes. Transfer to a large bowl and let cool for 10 minutes.

2. Preheat oven to 450 degrees F. Line a large rimmed baking sheet with foil and coat with cooking spray.

3. Add breadcrumbs, parsley, cheese, Italian seasoning, salt and pepper to the cooled vegetables; stir until combined. Add turkey and mix gently to combine (do not overmix). Form into 30 meatballs (a scant 2 tablespoons each) and place on the prepared baking sheet.

4. Bake the meatballs until an instant-read thermometer inserted in the center registers 165 degrees F, about 15 minutes.

Pizza Lettuce Wraps

Ingredients

- 1 ¼ cups cherry tomatoes or grape tomatoes, quartered

- ¾ cup shredded reduced-fat mozzarella cheese (3 ounces)

- 1 ounce thinly sliced, cooked turkey pepperoni, chopped (1/4 cup)

- ¼ cup snipped fresh basil

- 1 tablespoon snipped fresh oregano

- 8 large Bibb lettuce leaves

Directions

1. In a medium bowl combine tomatoes, cheese, pepperoni, basil, and oregano. Divide tomato mixture among lettuce leaves. Roll up or leave open as cups.

Reuben Pickle Bites

Ingredients

- 2 ½ tablespoons mayonnaise

- 1 tablespoon ketchup

- 1 teaspoon prepared horseradish

- ½ teaspoon Worcestershire sauce

- ¼ teaspoon onion powder

- 1-2 dashes hot sauce, such as Tabasco

- 2 tablespoons butter

- 2 medium slices rye bread, crusts trimmed, cut into 18 (1-inch) pieces

- 6 small slices pastrami or corned beef, cut into thirds (18 strips)

- 2 slices Swiss cheese, cut into 18 (1-inch) pieces

- 36 sliced kosher dill pickle rounds

Directions

1. Combine mayonnaise, ketchup, horseradish, Worcestershire, onion powder and hot sauce in a small bowl.

2. Heat butter in a large skillet over medium-high heat until melted. Add bread and cook, flipping once, until golden brown and crispy on both sides, 1 to 2 minutes per side.

3. To assemble bites: Onto each of 18 toothpicks, thread a pickle slice, a folded piece of pastrami (or corned beef), a piece of the bread and a piece of cheese. Add 1/2 teaspoon of the mayonnaise mixture and finish the skewer with another pickle slice.

Loaded Sweet Potato Nacho Fries

Ingredients

• 2 tablespoons extra-virgin olive oil

• 2 medium sweet potatoes (about 1 1/2 pounds), cut into sticks about 1/4 inch thick

• ¼ teaspoon salt plus a pinch, divided

• 2 tablespoons reduced-fat sour cream

• 1 tablespoon lime juice

• 1 cup corn kernels, fresh or frozen

• ½ cup shredded Cheddar cheese

• ⅓ cup black beans, rinsed

• ½ cup cherry tomatoes, halved or quartered if large

• 2 scallions, sliced

• 1 avocado, chopped

• 2 tablespoons chopped cilantro (Optional)

Directions

1. Preheat oven to 425 degrees F.

2. Heat oil in a large cast-iron skillet over medium-high heat. Add sweet potatoes and 1/4 teaspoon salt. Cook, stirring occasionally, until beginning to brown, 5 to 7 minutes. Transfer the pan to the oven and bake until the sweet potatoes are soft, 15 to 20 minutes.

3. Meanwhile, combine sour cream, lime juice and the remaining pinch of salt in a small bowl.

4. Top the sweet potatoes with corn, cheese and beans. Continue baking until the cheese is melted, about 5 minutes. Top with tomatoes, scallions and avocado. Drizzle with the sour cream mixture. Serve topped with cilantro (if using).

Fresh Tomato Salsa

Ingredients

• 4 cups diced tomatoes, (5-6 medium)

• 3/4 cup finely diced red onion, (about 1 small)

• ¼ cup red-wine vinegar

• 1-2 jalapenos, seeded and minced

• ½ cup chopped fresh cilantro

• ½ teaspoon salt

• Pinch of cayenne pepper, or more to taste

Directions

1. Combine tomatoes, onion, vinegar, jalapeno, cilantro, salt and cayenne in a medium bowl. Refrigerate until ready to serve.

Sicilian Caponata

Ingredients

- 6 tablespoons extra-virgin olive oil, divided

- 1 pound eggplant (see Tips), peeled and diced

- 1 large sweet onion, diced

- 2 cloves garlic, minced

- 3 stalks celery with leaves, diced

- 3 plum tomatoes, diced

- 1 tablespoon sugar, if needed

- 1 tablespoon red-wine or white-wine vinegar, or more to taste

- 1 teaspoon kosher salt

- Freshly ground pepper to taste

- 1 tablespoon capers, rinsed

- 2 tablespoons chopped fresh basil

• 15 small or 7 large pitted green olives, quartered

• 2 tablespoons lightly toasted pine nuts (see Tips)

Directions

1. Heat 4 tablespoons oil in a 12-inch nonstick skillet over medium heat. Add eggplant and cook, stirring occasionally, until lightly browned and soft, 5 to 10 minutes. Transfer to a plate.

2. Heat the remaining 2 tablespoons oil in the pan. Add onion and cook, stirring frequently, until soft and lightly golden, 6 to 8 minutes. Stir in garlic and cook, stirring, for 30 seconds. (If the pan seems too dry, push the onion and garlic to the side, add a drizzle of oil, then continue cooking.)

3. Stir in celery; cook, stirring frequently, until softened and slightly golden, 5 to 7 minutes. Stir in tomatoes; cook, stirring, about 2 minutes. Return the eggplant to the pan; stir until well combined. Sprinkle sugar over the eggplant mixture (omit if using Chinese eggplant, which is naturally sweeter), stir to combine and cook for about 30 seconds. Stir in vinegar, salt and pepper. Taste and add 1 to 2 tablespoons vinegar, if desired. Stir in olives and capers; cook for 1 minute. Remove the pan from the heat. Stir in basil and pine nuts.

Main Courses

Pesto Spaghetti Squash

Ingredients

• 1 spaghetti squash, halved lengthwise and seeded

• 3 tablespoons butter, divided

• 1 onion, sliced

• 1 cup kale, stems removed and leaves chopped

• 4 white mushrooms, sliced

• 1 teaspoon garlic salt

• 1 teaspoon Italian seasoning

• 1 teaspoon red pepper flakes

• 1 teaspoon olive oil

• 2 tablespoons prepared pesto

• ¼ cup grated Parmesan cheese

Directions

1. Preheat the oven to 400 degrees F (200 degrees C). Grease a baking sheet.

2. Place squash skin-side down on prepared baking sheet. Bake until cooked through, about 1 hour. Remove from oven; cool for 10 minutes. Once squash is cool enough to handle, scrape flesh into string-like strands with a fork. Place in a bowl and set aside.

3. Melt 1 tablespoon of butter in a large skillet over medium-high heat. Add onion; cook and stir until onion begins to turn translucent. Stir in kale and mushrooms; reduce heat to medium low.

4. Stir in squash, remaining 2 tablespoons butter, garlic salt, Italian seasoning, and red pepper flakes; cook for 2 minutes. Remove from stove and place squash mixture in a large bowl.

5. Stir olive oil and pesto into the squash mixture. Slowly add grated Parmesan cheese, stirring until evenly mixed.

Black Beans and Rice

Ingredients

• 1 teaspoon olive oil

• 1 onion, chopped

• 2 cloves garlic, minced

• ¾ cup uncooked white rice

• 1 ½ cups low sodium, low fat vegetable broth

- 3 ½ cups canned black beans, drained

- 1 teaspoon ground cumin

- ¼ teaspoon cayenne pepper

Directions

1. Heat oil in a saucepan over medium-high heat. Add onion and garlic; cook and stir until onion has softened, about 4 minutes. Stir in rice to coat; cook and stir for 2 minutes.

2. Add vegetable broth and bring to a boil. Cover, reduce to a simmer, and cook until liquid is absorbed, about 20 minutes.

3. Stir in beans, cumin, and cayenne; cook until beans are warmed through.

Veggie Pizza

Ingredients

- 2 (8 ounce) packages refrigerated crescent rolls

- 1 cup sour cream

- 1 (8 ounce) package cream cheese, softened

- 1 (1 ounce) package ranch seasoning mix

- 1 teaspoon dried dill weed

- ¼ teaspoon garlic salt

- 1 ½ cups chopped fresh broccoli

- ½ cup halved and thinly-sliced radishes

- 1 small onion, finely chopped

- 1 red bell pepper, chopped

- 1 carrot, grated

- 1 stalk celery, thinly sliced

Directions

1. Preheat the oven to 350 degrees F (175 degrees C). Spray a jelly roll pan with nonstick cooking spray.

2. Press crescent roll dough into the prepared jelly roll pan to form a crust. Let stand 5 minutes. Pierce with a fork.

3. Bake in the preheated oven until dough is fully cooked and golden brown, about 10 minutes. Let cool completely.

4. Combine sour cream, cream cheese, ranch seasoning mix, dill, and garlic salt in a medium mixing bowl. Spread the cream cheese mixture on top of cooled crust. Arrange broccoli, radish, onion, bell pepper, carrot, and celery on top of the cream cheese mixture.

5. Cover and let chill, 1 to 2 hours. Cut chilled pizza into 16 squares to serve.

Italian Sausage, Peppers, and Onions

Ingredients

- 6 (4 ounce) links sweet Italian sausage

- 2 tablespoons butter

- 1 medium yellow onion, sliced

- ½ medium red onion, sliced

- 4 cloves garlic, minced

- 1 large red bell pepper, sliced

- 1 medium green bell pepper, sliced

- 1 teaspoon dried basil

- 1 teaspoon dried oregano

- ¼ cup white wine, or more to taste

Directions

1. Cook sausage in a large skillet over medium heat until brown on all sides, 5 to 7 minutes. Remove from skillet, and slice.

2. Melt butter in the same skillet. Stir in onions and garlic, and cook 2 to 3 minutes. Mix in bell peppers, season with basil and oregano, and stir in 1/4 cup wine. Continue to cook and stir until peppers and onions are tender, 5 to 7 minutes.

3. Return sausage slices to the skillet. Reduce heat to low, cover, and simmer 15 minutes, or until sausage is heated through, adding more wine if needed.

4. Serve hot and enjoy!

Air Fryer Baked Potatoes

Ingredients

• 2 large russet potatoes, scrubbed

• 1 tablespoon peanut oil

• ½ teaspoon coarse sea salt

Directions

1. Preheat an air fryer to 400 degrees F (200 degrees C).

2. Brush potatoes with peanut oil, sprinkle with salt, and place them in the air fryer basket.

3. Cook potatoes until very tender when pierced with a fork, about 1 hour.

Salmon Rice Bowl

Ingredients

• 4 ounces salmon, preferably wild

- 1 teaspoon avocado oil

- ⅛ teaspoon kosher salt

- 1 cup instant brown rice

- 1 cup water

- 2 tablespoons mayonnaise

- 1 ½ teaspoons Sriracha

- 1 ½ teaspoons 50%-less-sodium tamari

- 1 teaspoon mirin

- ½ teaspoon freshly grated ginger

- ¼ teaspoon crushed red pepper

- ⅛ teaspoon kosher salt

- ½ ripe avocado, chopped

- ½ cup chopped cucumber

- ¼ cup spicy kimchi

- 12 (4-inch) sheets nori (roasted seaweed)

Directions

1. Preheat oven to 400ºF. Line a small rimmed baking sheet with foil. Place salmon on the prepared pan. Drizzle with oil; season with salt. Bake until an instant-read thermometer inserted in the thickest part registers 125ºF, 8 to 10 minutes.

2. Meanwhile, combine rice and water in a small saucepan; cook according to package directions. Mix mayonnaise and Sriracha in a small bowl; set aside. Whisk tamari, mirin, ginger, crushed red pepper and salt in another small bowl; set aside.

3. Divide the rice between 2 bowls. Top with salmon, avocado, cucumber and kimchi. Drizzle with the tamari mixture and the mayonnaise mixture. Mix the bowls, if desired, and serve with nori.

Spinach & Artichoke Dip Pasta

Ingredients

• 8 ounces whole-wheat rotini

• 1 (5 ounce) package baby spinach, roughly chopped

• 4 ounces reduced-fat cream cheese, cut into chunks

• ¾ cup reduced-fat milk

• ½ cup grated Parmesan cheese, plus more for garnish, if desired

• 2 teaspoons garlic powder

• ¼ teaspoon ground pepper

- 1 (14 ounce) can artichoke hearts, rinsed, squeezed dry and chopped (see Tip)

Directions

1. Bring a large saucepan of water to a boil. Cook pasta according to package directions. Drain.

2. Combine spinach and 1 tablespoon water in a large saucepan over medium heat. Cook, stirring occasionally, until just wilted, about 2 minutes. Transfer to a small bowl.

3. Add cream cheese and milk to the pan; whisk until the cream cheese is melted.

4. Add Parmesan, garlic powder and pepper; cook, whisking until thickened and bubbling.

5. Drain as much liquid as possible from the spinach. Stir the drained spinach into the sauce, along with artichokes and the pasta. Cook until warmed through.

Crab Louie Salad

Ingredients

Dressing

- ½ cup ketchup

- ½ cup mayonnaise

- ¼ cup minced yellow onion

- 1 clove garlic, minced

- 1 tablespoon dill pickle relish

- 2 teaspoons dried dill

- 1 teaspoon prepared horseradish

- 1 teaspoon lemon juice

Salad

- 8 asparagus spears, trimmed

- 1 medium head green-leaf lettuce, torn

- 2 medium tomatoes, cut into wedges

- 2 hard-boiled eggs, quartered

- 2 stalks celery, sliced

- 1 ripe avocado, sliced

- ½ medium cucumber, sliced

- 2 scallions, sliced

- ½ cup sliced canned pitted black olives, rinsed

- ¼ cup sliced red onion

- 6 ounces cooked crabmeat

• Lemon wedges for serving

Directions

1. To prepare dressing: Whisk ketchup, mayonnaise, yellow onion, garlic, relish, dill, horseradish and lemon juice in a medium bowl.

2. To prepare salad: Bring 1 inch of water to a boil in a large pot fitted with a steamer basket. Place a bowl of ice water near the stove. Add asparagus to the pot, cover and steam until tender-crisp, 3 to 5 minutes. Transfer to the ice bath. Drain and pat dry.

3. Place lettuce on a serving platter. Arrange the asparagus, tomatoes, eggs, celery, avocado, cucumber, scallions, olives and red onion on top. Top with crabmeat and dollop with half the dressing (reserve the remaining dressing for another use). Serve with lemon wedges, if desired.

Sides and Accompaniments

Zucchini Rice Casserole

Ingredients

- 1 1/2 cups long-grain brown rice

- 3 cups reduced-sodium chicken broth

- 4 cups diced zucchini , and/or summer squash (about 1 pound)

- 2 red or green bell peppers, chopped

- 1 large onion, diced

- ¾ teaspoon salt

- 1 1/2 cups low-fat milk

- 3 tablespoons all-purpose flour

- 2 cups shredded pepper Jack cheese, divided

- 1 cup fresh or frozen (thawed) corn kernels

- 2 teaspoons extra-virgin olive oil

- 8 ounces turkey sausage, casings removed

- 4 ounces reduced-fat cream cheese , (Neufchâtel)

- ¼ cup chopped pickled jalapeños

Directions

1. Preheat oven to 375 degrees F.

2. Pour rice into a 9-by-13-inch baking dish. Bring broth to a simmer in a small saucepan. Stir hot broth into the rice along with zucchini (and/or squash), bell peppers, onion and salt. Cover with foil. Bake for 45 minutes. Remove foil and continue baking until the rice is tender and most of the liquid is absorbed, 35 to 45 minutes more.

3. Meanwhile, whisk milk and flour in a small saucepan. Cook over medium heat until bubbling and thickened, 3 to 4 minutes. Reduce heat to low. Add 1 1/2 cups Jack cheese and corn and cook, stirring, until the cheese is melted. Set aside.

4. Heat oil in a large skillet over medium heat and add sausage. Cook, stirring and breaking the sausage into small pieces with a spoon, until lightly browned and no longer pink, about 4 minutes.

5. When the rice is done, stir in the sausage and cheese sauce. Sprinkle the remaining 1/2 cup Jack cheese on top and dollop cream cheese by the teaspoonful over the casserole. Top with jalapenos.

6. Return the casserole to the oven and bake until the cheese is melted, about 10 minutes. Let stand for about 10 minutes before serving.

Quinoa with Peas & Lemon

Ingredients

- 1 tablespoon extra-virgin olive oil

- 1 shallot, chopped

- 1 (10 ounce) package frozen peas

- 2 cups cooked quinoa

- Zest of 1 lemon

- ¼ cup crumbled goat cheese

- ¾ teaspoon salt

- ½ teaspoon ground pepper

Directions

1. Heat oil in a large skillet over medium-high heat. Add shallot and cook, stirring, until softened, about 2 minutes. Stir in peas and quinoa; cook, stirring often, until heated through, about 5 minutes. Stir in lemon zest, goat cheese, salt and pepper.

Nina's Mexican Rice

Ingredients

- 2 tablespoons canola oil

- 1 cup long-grain white rice (see Brown Rice Variation)

- ½ cup finely chopped onion

- ¼ teaspoon salt

- 1 tablespoon minced garlic

- 1 8-ounce can tomato sauce

- 1 1/2 cups reduced-sodium chicken broth or vegetable broth

- 1/2 cup frozen mixed vegetables (such as corn, peas and carrots), thawed

Directions

1. Heat a large heavy saucepan with a tight-fitting lid over medium heat. Add oil and rice and cook, stirring, until the rice is just beginning to brown, 4 to 5 minutes. Add onion and salt and cook, stirring, until the onion begins to soften, about 2 minutes. Add garlic and cook, stirring, until fragrant, 1 minute more. Pour tomato sauce over the rice and cook, stirring, for 1 minute.

2. Stir in broth and bring to a boil. Reduce to a simmer, cover and cook until the rice is cooked, about 15 minutes. Stir in vegetables and serve.

3. Brown Rice Variation: Use 1 cup long-grain brown rice and 1 3/4 cups broth. In Step 2, simmer for 45 minutes. Remove the rice from the heat and let stand, covered, for 15 minutes before adding the vegetables.

Savory Millet Cakes

Ingredients

• 1 tablespoon extra-virgin olive oil

• ¼ cup finely chopped onion

• 1 cup millet, (see Note)

• 1 clove garlic, minced

• 3 ½ cups water

• ½ teaspoon coarse salt

• ⅓ cup coarsely shredded zucchini

• ⅓ cup coarsely shredded carrot

• ⅓ cup grated Parmesan cheese

• 1 1/2 teaspoons minced fresh thyme, or 1/2 teaspoon dried

• 1 teaspoon freshly grated lemon zest

• ¼ teaspoon freshly ground pepper

Directions

1. Heat 1 tablespoon oil in a large saucepan over medium-low heat. Add onion and cook, stirring, until softened, 2 to 4 minutes. Stir in millet and garlic and cook, stirring, until fragrant, about 30 seconds. Add water and salt and bring to a boil

over medium heat. Reduce heat to low, cover and cook, stirring once or twice, for 20 minutes. Stir in zucchini, carrot, Parmesan, thyme, lemon zest and pepper. Cook, uncovered, maintaining a simmer and stirring often to keep the millet from sticking, until the mixture is soft, very thick and the liquid has been absorbed, about 10 minutes more. Remove from the heat and let stand, covered, for 10 minutes. Uncover and let stand, stirring once or twice, until cool enough to handle, about 30 minutes.

2. With dampened hands, shape the millet mixture into 12 cakes or patties, 3-inch diameter (a scant 1/3 cup each).

3. Coat a large nonstick skillet with cooking spray and heat over medium heat. Add 4 millet cakes and cook until the bottoms are browned, 3 to 5 minutes. Carefully turn the cakes with a wide spatula and cook until the other side is browned, 3 to 5 minutes more. Coat the pan with cooking spray again and cook the remaining cakes in batches, reducing the heat if necessary to prevent burning.

Eggplant Caponata

Ingredients

• 2 pounds eggplant, peeled and cut into 1/2-inch cubes

• 1 tablespoon sea salt

• ½ cup extra-virgin olive oil, divided

- 3 bay leaves

- 1 pound onions, chopped

- 1 pound celery, sliced 1/2-inch thick

- 1 pound cherry tomatoes, halved

- ¼ cup capers, preferably salt-packed, well rinsed

- 20 large green olives, pitted and very coarsely chopped

- 2 fresh hot red chile peppers, halved, seeded and thinly sliced

- ½ cup red-wine vinegar

- 1 tablespoon honey

- 2 tablespoons chopped flat-leaf parsley

- 2 tablespoons chopped fresh basil

Directions

1. Combine eggplant and salt in a large bowl. Transfer to a colander, place a plate on the eggplant and weigh down the plate with cans. Set the colander in the sink to drain for 1 hour.

2. Meanwhile, heat 1/4 cup oil in a large skillet over medium heat. Add bay leaves and let sizzle for about 1 minute to flavor the oil. Stir in onions and celery. Reduce heat to medium-low; cook, stirring occasionally, until the vegetables are soft, about 30 minutes (do not let them brown). Add tomatoes and capers; increase

heat to medium and cook, stirring occasionally, just until the tomatoes start to break down, about 5 minutes. Stir in olives; transfer the mixture to a large bowl.

3. When the eggplant is ready, rinse under running water to get rid of as much salt as possible. Dry thoroughly on paper towels.

4. Heat the remaining 1/4 cup oil in the same skillet over medium heat until very hot. Add the eggplant; cook, tossing and stirring, until brown on all sides, 10 to 15 minutes. Add chiles; cook, stirring, until softened, 5 to 10 minutes. Transfer the eggplant and chiles to the bowl with the tomato mixture; gently stir to combine.

5. Whisk vinegar and honey in a small saucepan; bring to a boil over medium heat. Simmer until thickened and reduced to about 1/4 cup, about 5 minutes. Stir into the vegetables along with parsley and basil. Serve at room temperature.

Sesame Cucumber Salad

Ingredients

• 1 Japanese cucumber or 4 Persian mini cucumbers (about 10 ounces)

• 2 tablespoons rice vinegar

• 1 tablespoon toasted sesame oil

• ¼ teaspoon grated garlic

• ¼ teaspoon grated ginger

- ⅛ teaspoon salt

- Pinch of sugar

- 1 teaspoon sesame seeds

Directions

1. Peel cucumber to leave alternating green stripes. Quarter the cucumber lengthwise (halve lengthwise if using Persian cucumbers) and cut into 1/2-inch slices. Pat with a paper towel to remove any excess moisture.

2. Whisk vinegar, sesame oil, garlic, ginger and salt in a medium bowl. Add the cucumber slices and toss to coat. Serve topped with sesame seeds.

Roasted Savoy Cabbage with Pistachios & Lemon

Ingredients

- 1 (1 1/2-pound) head savoy cabbage, cored and cut into 1- to 2-inch pieces

- 3 tablespoons extra-virgin olive oil

- 1 teaspoon ground coriander

- ½ teaspoon salt

- ½ teaspoon ground pepper

- ½ teaspoon grated lemon zest

• 1 tablespoon lemon juice

• ¼ cup chopped unsalted roasted pistachios

Directions

1. Preheat oven to 425°F. Toss cabbage with oil, coriander, salt and pepper on a large rimmed baking sheet. Roast, stirring halfway through, until tender and golden brown in places, about 25 minutes.

2. Stir in lemon zest, lemon juice and pistachios.

Soups and Salads

Beet Salad with Goat Cheese

Ingredients

• 4 medium beets - scrubbed, trimmed, and cut in half

• 1/3 cup chopped walnuts

• 3 tablespoons maple syrup

• 1 (10 ounce) package mixed baby salad greens

• 1/2 cup frozen orange juice concentrate

• 1/4 cup balsamic vinegar

• 1/2 cup extra-virgin olive oil

• 2 ounces goat cheese

Directions

1. Place beets into a saucepan; add enough water to cover. Bring to a boil, then cook for 20 to 30 minutes, until tender. Drain and cool, then cut into cubes.

2. While beets are cooking, place walnuts in a skillet over medium-low heat. Heat until warm and starting to toast. Stir in maple syrup; cook and stir until evenly coated, then remove from heat and set aside to cool.

3. To make the dressing: Whisk orange juice concentrate, balsamic vinegar, and olive oil together in a small bowl.

4. Place a large helping of baby greens onto each of four salad plates, divide candied walnuts equally and sprinkle over greens. Place equal amounts of beets over greens and top with pieces of goat cheese. Drizzle dressing over each salad.

Old-Fashioned Potato Salad

Ingredients

• 5 potatoes

• 3 eggs

• 1 cup chopped celery

• ½ cup chopped onion

• ½ cup sweet pickle relish

• ¼ cup mayonnaise

• 1 tablespoon prepared mustard

• ¼ teaspoon garlic salt

• ¼ teaspoon celery salt

• ground black pepper to taste

Directions

1. Gather all ingredients.

2. Bring a large pot of salted water to a boil. Add potatoes and cook until tender but still firm, about 15 minutes.

3. Drain, cool, peel, and chop potatoes.

4. While potatoes cook, place eggs in a saucepan and cover with cold water. Bring water to a boil; cover, remove from heat, and let eggs stand in hot water for 10 to 12 minutes.

5. Remove from hot water, cool, peel, and chop eggs.

6. Combine the potatoes, eggs, celery, onion, relish, mayonnaise, mustard, garlic salt, celery salt, and pepper in a large bowl. Mix together well and refrigerate until chilled.

7. Enjoy!

Bodacious Broccoli Salad

Ingredients

• 8 slices bacon

• 2 heads fresh broccoli, chopped

• 1 ½ cups sharp Cheddar cheese, shredded

- ½ large red onion, chopped

- ⅔ cup mayonnaise

- ¼ cup red wine vinegar

- ⅛ cup white sugar

- 2 teaspoons ground black pepper

- 1 teaspoon salt

- 1 teaspoon fresh lemon juice

Directions

1. Place bacon in a large, deep skillet. Cook over medium-high heat until crisp and evenly browned, 8-10 minutes. Transfer to a paper towel-lined plate and crumble when cool enough to handle.

2. Combine bacon, broccoli, cheese, and onion in a large bowl.

3. Whisk mayonnaise, red wine vinegar, sugar, pepper, salt, and lemon juice together in a small bowl; pour over salad and toss to combine. Cover and refrigerate until ready to serve.

Cauliflower Gruyere Soup

Ingredients

- 8 cups coarsely chopped cauliflower

- 2 tablespoons olive oil

- 1 ⅓ cups low-sodium vegetable broth, or more as needed

- ¼ teaspoon salt

- ¼ teaspoon ground black pepper

- ¼ teaspoon garlic powder

- ½ cup heavy whipping cream

- 6 tablespoons shredded Gruyere cheese

- 1 tablespoon chopped fresh parsley, or to taste

Directions

1. Preheat oven to 425 degrees F (220 degrees C). Line a baking sheet with foil.

2. Toss together cauliflower and oil in a bowl. Spread cauliflower on the prepared baking sheet in a single layer.

3. Roast, stirring once, until cauliflower is tender and just starting to brown, about 30 minutes. (Do not overbrown cauliflower or it will become bitter.) Reserve 1/2 cup florets for garnish and keep warm. Let remaining cauliflower cool slightly.

4. Combine cooled roasted cauliflower 1 1/3 cups broth, salt, pepper, and garlic powder in blender or food processor, working in batches, if needed. Cover and blend until smooth, adding more broth as needed to reach desired consistency.

5. Transfer mixture to a saucepan. Bring just to a boil over medium heat. Remove from heat. Stir in cream and 2 tablespoons cheese until melted. Serve topped with reserved cauliflower florets, remaining cheese, the parsley, and if you like, additional pepper.

Easy Spinach Soup

Ingredients

• 2 ½ tablespoons butter

• ½ cup chopped carrots

• ½ cup chopped scallions

• 1 clove garlic, minced

• 6 cups chicken broth

• ½ cup orzo

• 1 (10 ounce) bag fresh spinach, chopped

• salt and ground black pepper to taste

Directions

1. Melt butter in a stockpot over medium heat. Add carrots, scallions, and garlic; cook and stir until scallions are soft, 1 to 2 minutes. Pour in chicken broth; bring to a boil.

2. Add pasta and cook, stirring occasionally until tender yet firm to the bite, 5 to 10 minutes. Stir in spinach; cook until tender, 2 to 3 minutes more. Season with salt and pepper.

Classic Vichyssoise

Ingredients

• 1 tablespoon butter

• 3 leeks, bulb only, sliced into rings

• 1 onion, sliced

• 5 medium potatoes, peeled and thinly sliced

• salt and pepper to taste

• ½ teaspoon dried marjoram

• ¼ teaspoon dried thyme

• 1 bay leaf

• 5 cups chicken broth

• ¼ cup heavy whipping cream

Directions

1. Melt butter in a large stockpot over low heat. Add leeks and onion; cover and cook for 10 minutes.

2. Stir in potatoes; season with salt and pepper. Add marjoram, thyme, and bay leaf; stir well. Cover and cook for 12 minutes.

3. Pour in chicken broth. Bring to a boil, reduce heat, and cook, partially covered, for 30 minutes.

4. Purée soup in a blender or food processor. Allow to cool to room temperature, then stir in cream.

French Onion Soup Gratinée

Ingredients

• 4 tablespoons butter

• 2 large red onions, thinly sliced

• 2 large sweet onions, thinly sliced

• 1 teaspoon salt

• 1 (48 fluid ounce) can chicken broth

- 1 (14 ounce) can beef broth

- ½ cup red wine

- 1 tablespoon Worcestershire sauce

- 2 sprigs fresh parsley

- 1 sprig fresh thyme leaves

- 1 bay leaf

- 1 tablespoon balsamic vinegar

- salt and freshly ground black pepper to taste

- 4 thick slices French bread

- 8 slices Gruyère cheese, at room temperature

- ½ cup shredded Asiago cheese, at room temperature

- 4 pinches paprika

Directions

1. Melt butter in a large pot over medium-high heat. Stir in red onions, sweet onions, and salt. Cook, stirring frequently, until onions are caramelized and almost syrupy, about 35 minutes.

2. Stir in chicken broth, beef broth, red wine, and Worcestershire sauce. Bundle parsley, thyme, and bay leaf with kitchen twine; add to the pot. Simmer over

medium heat for 20 minutes, stirring occasionally. Remove and discard herb bundle. Reduce heat to low; stir in vinegar and season with salt and pepper. Cover soup and keep warm over low heat while you prepare the toast.

3. Set an oven rack about 6 inches from the heat source and preheat the oven's broiler. Arrange bread slices on a baking sheet and broil, turning once, until well toasted on both sides, about 3 minutes. Remove from heat; do not turn off the broiler.

4. Arrange 4 large oven-safe bowls or crocks on a rimmed baking sheet. Fill each bowl 2/3 full with hot soup. Top each bowl with 1 slice of toasted bread, 2 slices Gruyère cheese, and 1/4 of the Asiago cheese. Sprinkle a little bit of paprika over the top of each one.

5. Cook under the hot broiler until bubbly and golden brown, about 5 minutes. Cheese will cascade over the sides of the crock and form a beautifully melted crusty seal as it melts.

6. Serve hot and enjoy!

Weekly Meal Plans and Shopping Lists

Day One

Breakfast

Tomato & Scrambled Egg on Low FODMAP Sourdough: 1 slice of low FODMAP sourdough bread topped with tomato + 2 scrambled eggs + cheddar cheese.

1 glass calcium-fortified rice or oat milk.

Lunch

Chicken and Quinoa Salad: 100g grilled chicken breast+ 1 cup cooked quinoa + 1 cup kale + tomato + red capsicum + ¼ cup mint + ground coriander and lemon juice.

Dinner

Tofu & Edamame Buddha Bowl: Made with 170g firm tofu+ 1/2 cup boiled edamame+ ¾ cup cabbage+ cucumber+ 2 slices haloumi (40g)+ 1 cup cooked brown rice+ 2tbsp tahini + 1tsp salt reduced soy sauce.

Dessert/Supper

Strawberries & Yoghurt Parfait: ¾ cup lactose-free yoghurt layered with 1 cup diced strawberries and 2tbsp sunflower seeds.

Snacks

1 medium orange + a handful of walnuts (30g)

Day Two

Breakfast

Vanilla Polenta Porridge with Strawberry: Made with 1/3 cup instant polenta mixed with 1 cup lactose-free milk + 2 tsp vanilla bean paste, cooked for 3-5 minutes, topped with walnuts, sunflower seeds & cinnamon. Add 4 strawberries.

Lunch

Tuna Salad: 1 canned tuna + 20g crumbled fetta cheese+ ½ cup canned corn kernels, ½ cup canned beetroot, carrot, lettuce, cucumber, tomato, with olive oil and lemon dressing. Served with low FODMAP bread.

+ bundle of grapes + a tub of yoghurt

Dinner

Grilled Steak with Vegetables: 1 medium grilled steak (using canola or olive oil) with 1 cup mashed potato and 2 cups roasted vegetables (red capsicum, baby corn, oyster mushroom, tomato).

Dessert/Supper

Fruit Salad: 1 cup of mixed fruit (grapes, strawberries, pineapple) + 2 tbsp walnuts.

Snacks

3 rice crispbread with 40g tasty cheese and sliced cucumber.

Day Three

Breakfast

Low FODMAP Breakfast Cereal & Fruit: 2/3 cup low FODMAP cereal + 1 cup calcium-fortified rice or oat milk, 1 tbsp linseeds,1tbsp chopped walnuts and a bundle of grapes.

Lunch

Bubble and Squeak Turkey Fritters with Poached Eggs(1.5 serve) —Use rice flour of low FODMAP plain flour.

Dinner

Chicken Risotto: 1 cup cooked risotto rice made with low FODMAP chicken/ vegetable stock + 3 pieces semi-dried tomatoes + ½ cup diced oyster mushroom + 100g chicken breast + basil leaves+ 1 tsp olive oil + salt & pepper to taste.

+ 2 cup side salad (e.g. cucumber, lettuce, carrots, red capsicum) with 1 tsp olive oil dressing.

Dessert/Supper

Frozen Yoghurt with Fruit: Serve strawberries and 60g raspberries with frozen lactose-free yoghurt.

Snacks

Rice crackers with 40g cheddar cheese.

Day four

Breakfast

Healthy French Toast (1 serve) served with 2 slices of low FODMAP/ GF bread.

+ 1 glass of lactose-free milk + 2 small kiwifruit.

Lunch

Lentil, Tomato and Kale Soup: Make soup with 1 cup cooked/ canned lentils with 1 cup canned tomato + 1 cup chopped kale +1 cup carrot + 1 tbsp pine nuts + low FODMAP vegetable stock + coriander + chilli powder (optional),

Serve with low FODMAP bread.

Dinner

Baked Salmon with Quinoa & Vegetables: 1 medium salmon fillet (120g), baked & served with 1 cup cooked quinoa + feta cheese+ 2 cups cooked vegetables (e.g. carrots, kale, red capsicum, ½ cup sweet potato) + 2 tsp oil in cooking or as a dressing with lemon juice.

Dessert/Supper

Papaya Sorbet: Freeze 1 cup papaya for 4-5 hours. Blend with ¼ cup hot water in food processor until smooth + 1tbsp lime juice and 1 tbsp walnuts.

Snacks

1 glass calcium-fortified rice or oat milk.

Day Five

Breakfast

Fruit Smoothie: Made with 6 strawberries and 2 small kiwifruit + 1 cup calcium-fortified rice or oat milk + 2 tsp chia seeds + 1 tbsp sunflower seeds + topped with ¼ cup Low FODMAP muesli.

Lunch

Egg, Lettuce and Tomato Sandwich: Made with 2 slices low FODMAP bread, 2 hard-boiled eggs, sliced tomato,1 slice 20g hard cheese and lettuce + 1 tbsp mayonnaise.

Dinner

Greek-style Egg Lemon Soup with Chicken and Greens(1.5 serve) using low FODMAP pasta and chicken stock.

+ 2 cup side salad (e.g. cucumber, lettuce, carrots, red capsicum) with 1 tsp olive oil dressing.

Dessert/Supper

Frozen Fruit: e.g. 1 cup grapes, 140g chopped pineapple, or 2 small kiwifruit.

+ Handful of walnuts (30g)

Snacks

1 tub lactose-free yoghurt

Day Six

Breakfast

Low FODMAP Muesli with Yoghurt & Fruit: ½ cup low FODMAP muesli + 1 tub lactose free yoghurt + 1 medium orange

Lunch

Chicken, Cheese & Salad Wrap: 100g chicken breast + 20g crumbled fetta cheese + 2 cup salad vegetables (e.g. lettuce, rocket, cucumber, carrot, red capsicum, tomato) rolled up in low FODMAP wrap.

+2 small mandarins

Dinner

Beef Stir fry with Rice Noodle: Stir fry 100g lean beef strips with 2 cups vegetables (e.g. carrot, oyster mushroom, red capsicum, cabbage, cucumber) + 1 cup cooked rice noodles + 2 tsp sesame oil for cooking.,

Dessert/Supper

Chia Pudding: Mix well together 3 tbsp chia seeds with 1 cup calcium-fortified rice or oat milk, refrigerate for 3-4 hours, topped with cinnamon, walnuts and 1 tbsp linseeds.

Snacks

Baked Kale Chips and a handful of walnuts (30g)

Day Seven

Breakfast

Ricotta & Fruit Wrap:1 slice of low FODMAP tortilla with ¼ cup ricotta, 1/3 sliced banana + ½ cup strawberries. Roll up into a wrap. + 1 glass lactose-free milk.

Lunch

Grilled White Fish & Vegetables: 1 medium piece grilled white fish with 2 cups steamed FODMAP friendly vegetables (e.g kale, silverbeet, carrot). Served with mashed potato. + 1 tub of lactose-free yoghurt.

Shopping List

Low FODMAP Vegetables

When it comes to vegetables, the amount of FODMAPs often depends on the portion size. While some veggies can be eaten freely without worrying about FODMAPS at all, others like broccoli or butternut squash can be consumed in smaller amounts. Below is a list of low FODMAP vegetables you can eat freely and those you have to watch maximum portion sizes with (as per Monash University app).

Vegetables To Enjoy Freely

• Bamboo shoots (canned or fresh)

• Bean sprouts

• Red bell pepper (capsicum)

• Chili pepper (green)

• Corn (baby, canned)

• Cucumber

• Ginger root

• Kale

• Kohlrabi

• Leafy greens/lettuces: Arugula (rocket), Butter lettuce, endive, iceberg lettuce, Red leaf lettuce, Romaine lettuce, watercress

• Dark leafy greens: collard greens, spinach (English) and Swiss chard

• Mushrooms (oyster)

• Green onions (scallions, tops only)

• Root vegetables: carrots, parsnips, potatoes (white), rutabaga (swedes), yams

• Radish

• Seaweed

• Spaghetti squash

• Tomatillo, tomato (Canned), tomato (Common)

• Water chestnuts

Low FODMAP Fruit

Many fruits are FODMAP-friendly. However, unlike most elimination diets, there are a few invisible factors at play making others very high in FODMAPS – sorbitol and excess fructose. These fruits are low in both, giving them the green light.

• Banana (unripe) or banana chips, plantains

• Citrus fruits: clementines, lemons, limes and oranges

- Coconut (shredded)

- Dragon fruit

- Durian

- Grapes

- Kiwifruit

- Papaya

- Passionfruit

- Pears

- Pineapple

- Plantains

- Rhubarb

- Starfruit

- Strawberries

- Tamarind

Low FODMAP Bread Choices

Try buckwheat, gluten-free bread, millet, oatmeal/flour, pumpernickel bread, quinoa, rye bread, spelt, sourdough bread.

Low FODMAP pasta options and alternatives

Try chickpea pasta, gluten-free pasta, quinoa pasta, spelt sourdough pasta, wheat sourdough pasta.

Low FODMAP cheese

Most cheese is low FODMAP due to its high-fat content and low carb content. High amounts of ricotta or paneer can be triggering, but almost all cheeses are a green light especially in a low to moderate dose.

Brie cheese, cream cheese, goat cheese, gruyere cheese, halloumi cheese, Havarti cheese, manchego cheese, Monterey jack cheese, mozzarella cheese, Pecorino Romano cheese, Swiss cheese.

• Paneer cheese (consume less than 2 cups)

• Ricotta cheese (consume less than ¾ cup)

Low FODMAP cereal options

With cereal, it is important to refer to the app which will list specific brand names of cereal or refer to the individual ingredients. Considering the abundance of commercial cereals, it's really on a case-by-case basis. However, there are a few safe bets...if carbs or sugar are not something you're trying to avoid.

• Corn flakes, Frosted Flakes (not super healthy though), Rice Puffs, Rice Krispies, Special K are okay.

Low FODMAP sweeteners

Brown sugar, coconut sugar, icing sugar (powdered sugar), maple syrup, palm sugar, raw sugar, rice malt syrup, stevia, white sugar. Avoid agave syrup and honey.

Low FODMAP baking ingredients

All sweeteners mentioned above, arrowroot flour, buckwheat flour, butter, cacao powder, cocoa powder, coconut flour, coconut milk powder, cornflour, corn starch, dark chocolate, eggs, gluten-free flour, green banana flour, millet flour, quinoa flour, rice flour, sorghum flour, spelt flour, teff flour. Avoid too much almond meal.

Low FODMAP condiments

Barbeque sauce, capers, chimichurri sauce (without garlic), chutney (check for onion), fish sauce, horseradish, jam and jellies of low-FODMAP fruits e.g. raspberry, strawberry, tamarind, mayonnaise, mint jelly and sauce, mustard, peanut butter, salsa verde (without garlic), salsa (without garlic/onion), shrimp paste, soy sauce, sriracha (low amounts), sweet and sour sauce, tomato sauce and paste, Vegemite, vinegar (all varieties except balsamic), wasabi, Worcestershire sauce. Some of these might contain a little garlic or onion however if the amount used is small (e.g. 1 tbsp), these might not cause any symptoms.

Low FODMAP drinks

You can still have coffee and alcohol while avoiding high-FODMAP foods – just make sure to double-check. The same goes for tea, but most varieties are going to be perfectly fine. You may want to avoid certain herbal teas and investigate individual ingredients to determine the FODMAP content.

Almond milk, beer, coffee (black), cranberry juice, drinking chocolate, Espresso, gin, hemp milk, kvass, lactose-free milk, macadamia milk, rice milk, sweetened condensed milk, tea (black, dandelion, green, liquorice, peppermint, rooibos, white), vodka, wheatgrass juice/powder, whiskey, wine (most varieties).

Made in the USA
Middletown, DE
07 July 2023

34698418R00051